The ABC to Zen Guide
to Health & Happiness

The ABC to Zen Guide to Health & Happiness

ROBERT EVAN TROP

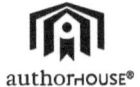

authorHOUSE®

AuthorHouse™
1663 Liberty Drive
Bloomington, IN 47403
www.authorhouse.com
Phone: 1-800-839-8640

First published by AuthorHouse 5/18/2010

ISBN: 978-1-4490-5059-7 (e)
ISBN: 978-1-4490-5058-0 (sc)

Library of Congress Control Number: 2010904305

Printed in the United States of America
Bloomington, Indiana

This book is printed on acid-free paper.

Acknowledgment

Many thanks go to my father, Milton Marc Trop, a brilliant man who still inspires me with his pursuit of knowledge and healthy, positive living habits. The "ABC" idea for this book actually came from something he said one day, reciting off a few items under an "ABC" rubric about some simple rules for staying healthy. He is eighty now and still plays tennis whenever the weather permits. My father's "ABC" items were a little different than those in this book, and he only covered the first seven letters or so of the alphabet.

I started making a list of "ABC" items in my spare time, and then I thought: *Why not cover the entire alphabet?* The idea intrigued me, and I decided to put it into a permanent form based on my own knowledge, research, experiences, and observations, which resulted in this book. I hope you enjoy reading it as much as I enjoyed writing it.

Dedication

For Luz Aida, my Lady of the Light, who is such a wonderful, healthy spirit and who inspires me to live healthy every day in every way possible.

Also by Robert Evan Trop

Leaves of Memory CD (2009) available on iTunes, CDBaby.com, Napster, and other music sites.

www.robertevantrop.com

How to Use This Book

For many people, the achievement of a healthy lifestyle remains elusive. There are many reasons good health seems rarer than ever for so many people; however, good health is possible to obtain, and the ways to do so are quite simple.

For this reason, this book is partially an aspirational book. In a perfect world, however, the behavior it outlines might be the way everyone could live for themselves and others.

Perhaps some of the information contained in this book will cause people to change their unhealthy dietary, physical, and mental/emotional lifestyle choices, all of which contribute to poor health.

When you are deciding how to be physically and emotionally healthy, you have to learn not to just accept what is offered to you, whether it is food or emotional conflict. You must learn how to make choices that benefit your physical and emotional health.

Just because something is does not mean it should be so, as it relates to you and your choices. Stated another way, just because you can do something does not mean that you should. Use your mind and the beauty of free will to make good, positive choices that will make you a more healthy and happy person.

"Life is a sum of all your choices."

—*ALBERT CAMUS*

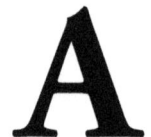

Alkaline

What does this mean? Do you remember your biology class in high school? "Alkaline" and "acidic" are terms used to address the state of liquid solutions on the pH scale. When your body is acidic, it is prone to disease. The obvious disease is cancer, a disease caused by cells that mutate primarily because of an acidic body condition. This disease is the most diet-related disease ever, and it is why there has never been and most likely never will be a real cure. There are many other diseases that are also primarily diet related, namely heart disease and diabetes, two of the most common.

What makes your body acidic? Your diet does. *Think* about what you eat. Basically, fruits, beans, nuts, vegetables, and water help make or return your body to an alkaline state. *Everything else* for the most part promotes an acidic condition. If your body becomes acidic, you should try to return it to an alkaline condition. If your body is constantly acidic, you will be more prone to sickness and eventually serious diseases, especially cancer.

Keep in your mind that your body was *not* designed to eat cooked meats, processed meats, manufactured sugar and sugar products, or bread products.

Processed and manufactured foods are the worst things you can put into your body. There are a myriad of manufactured and processed foods, which you are presented with every day, that have additives and chemicals your body does not need nor was designed to process at a cellular level. Keep this in mind as you eat. Try to limit those items when you can, and think of balancing any foods that create an acidic state with those that promote an alkaline state.

White sugar is a carcinogen. Any food with white sugar should be avoided or at least limited as much as possible, so be conscious of this fact. Drinking a lot of coffee and tea with lots of sugar may be tempting, but this will definitely leave you susceptible to cancer and other diseases as well. Soda and other artificially sweetened drinks, including so-called "energy drinks," are drinks that your body was definitely not designed to metabolize.

B

Blood Pressure

High blood pressure will ruin your blood vessels, damage your kidneys, make you prone to heart attacks, strokes, and cause other health problems over time. The narrowing of blood vessels is largely related to diet and stress. Incidentally, salt should not be completely eliminated from your diet.

Salt helps keep your body alkaline, which is important in preventing cells from mutating into cancer cells. Remember, if your body is alkaline, cancer cannot form. You will naturally have salt in your system if you have a proper diet. You should never add salt to food that is ready to eat. This is one of the problems with eating out. When food is prepared at restaurants, it often is oversalted before it gets to the table.

With a proper diet, exercise, stress elimination (or management), and proper water intake, you should not have high blood pressure. If the amount of salt in your body is too high, drinking enough water is critical, as water helps flush excess salt (as well as toxins) out of your body.

C

Children

Children can complicate your life in many stressful ways, thus compromising your health. Your physical health is related to your mental health and vice versa. They are, in fact, deeply connected. Bringing children into this world is a huge mental, physical, and financial undertaking, and once they are here, you are obligated to provide for them in a plethora of ways.

In modern society, it can be quite difficult to manage parenthood and your other obligations such as work. Moreover, you need time for *yourself* if you are to maintain your mental health. Before you start having children, you should think about where you are in life's journey and the years of stress you will have raising children. It is not okay to have children at any time in life. Remember, you never stop being a parent.

Cholesterol

Cholesterol is something you should keep to a minimum, and it relates to the previous category of blood pressure. Once again, you need to think about the foods that are high in cholesterol. Eating naturally (e.g., nuts, beans, fruits, and vegetables), drinking an adequate amount of water, and exercising regularly will eliminate this problem or at least temper it significantly.

No individual should have high cholesterol. Your mindset should not be that you will simply take a prescription medication. If your diet is proper, and you are not sedentary, you will not have high cholesterol—or high blood pressure—it is as simple as that.

Computer

The computer is a great source of information, but it has a dark side, because it will distract you with irrelevant things that waste your valuable time. Time is one of the most precious things in life, and you and only you should decide how to spend your time. Try to use your time wisely and productively.

Spending a lot of time in front of the computer can lead to fatigue. It can affect your ability to manage stress and make good decisions. Fatigue can also affect your moral and mental clarity, both of which affect your overall happiness. The computer is the modern day equivalent of the television. You should try to turn it off more often. There are better ways to spend your time that will make you a happier person.

Conflicts

You must know when to let things go to avoid unnecessary conflicts with other people. Conflict adds to your stress, which will weaken your physical health. You might consider applying Newton's third law when you are deciding how to interact with other people when there may be a conflict.

Newton stated as follows: *"For every action there is an equal and opposite reaction."* Consider that statement when you deal with people. Acting aggressive toward them will only increase the chance that they will react with negative words or actions against you, adding to your stress.

Consequences

All of your decisions ultimately affect your physical health (e.g., dietary choices and decisions that affect your physical safety), your emotional health (as a result of your stress level), and just as importantly, the health of those around you. Every decision you make—from what you eat to your thoughts to your lifestyle choices—has consequences.

This is especially true when decisions you make affect your children. Bad decisions and behaviors will forever affect your children, whether concerning bad dietary choices, alcohol, or drug abuse. Try to be aware of the potential effects your decisions have on yourself and those around you, whether those effects are direct or indirect.

D

Desire

Desire for your mate is important to your well-being. Keep this in mind so that you don't just marry a person who fits into a certain social strata or so that you don't marry someone to appease your parents or family histories. If you don't have desire for your mate, you are dooming yourself to eventual resentfulness, with the likelihood of developing a strong desire to pursue relations with a different person.

Diet

See "Alkaline" on p. 5.

E

Electromagnetic Radiation

We are exposed to electromagnetic radiation almost every day from all types of electronic devices, such as computers, televisions, cell phones, among numerous other devices. This is problematic because of the proximity of these devices to our bodies. When using these devices so close the body (especially cell phones and laptop computers placed on your lap), you are exposing yourself to levels of electromagnetic frequencies (EMF) that can damage your cells from repeated exposure.

EMF contributes to the alteration of cell structures. As such, this can become part of the cancer equation. If your body is also toxic (i.e., acidic), you are more likely to develop cancer. (See the related section of "Alkaline" on p. 5.)

Some people's genetic makeup makes them less susceptible to cell mutation. Everyone is not created equal in this regard. Unless you know that your body is superhuman—of course, no one is—and is not affected by EMF, then you should at least bear this point in mind. Try to limit your exposure to devices that emit EMF by avoiding close proximity and prolonged exposure to them on a regular basis.

Employment

Where you work and kind of work you do will have a tremendous effect on your health. Stress is one of the biggest by-products of your job, and years of job stress will take a toll on your mental health, which will in turn affect your physical well-being. Do not be afraid to change your employment for this reason.

The type of job a person does tends to also affect a person's dietary choices during the day. After eating poorly for breakfast (typically for time reasons or just poor dietary habits), many people then compound their daily unhealthy eating with an unhealthy lunch. Thereafter, people often add to their body's poor cellular nutrition, and make themselves even more toxic by snacking at work on manufactured foods.

All manufactured foods are, as a general rule, unhealthy, due to chemicals, artifical substances, and other items your body was not designed to metabolize either for digestion or for cellular energy. Making matters worse for your overall health is the fact that many jobs, if not most of them, call for people to sit most of the day.

Excessive sitting promotes weight gain and other health problems. This is because the human animal was not supposed to spend many hours during the day sitting.

Your level of job satisfaction also stems from what you do. Do you help people? Do you merely do what you do to make money for yourself or some artificial entity such as a corporation? True satisfaction comes from helping others.

Your job, which comprises a huge chunk of your waking life, is keyed into your true satisfaction. True satisfaction in turn is keyed into your mental health, which in turn is keyed into your physical health.

Exercise

One of the most important things in maintaining your body's functioning is exercise or physical activity. The more natural the exercise, the better it is for you. The human body was not designed to play many of the sports created by man, or to endure the repetitive or physically strenuous exercises that many people subject their bodies to.

This is why people routinely injure their muscles, tear tendons and soft cartilage, and end up with body parts with a greatly shortened useful lifespan. These body parts literally "wear out" before their time due to improper use and overuse. Surgery may be an option; however, the body is like a car. As a general principle, once it is damaged, it will never be the same.

One of the best exercises you can do is walking. It is low impact and elevates your mental mood, because it releases hormones that promote feeling good. Bear in mind that while you can exercise in a more strenuous way, you should always ask yourself if you are overdoing it. While you may get away with it while you are young, it will only be a matter of time before you injure yourself.

F

Faith

Having faith that there is some greater good beyond your own is a positive notion. It is healthy for your mind because it fosters hope, a healthy mental state.

Forgiveness

In your heart as in every person's heart is the ability to forgive. Holding grudges and being angry only leads to hateful thoughts and ideas. Hate is one of the Three Poisons of the Mind that leads to an unhealthy emotional state. (See the section "Poisons of the Mind" on p. 47.)

Friends

The human animal is meant to form relationships and interact with people. Look to form friendships with different types of people who will be a positive influence on you. Don't limit yourself to friends who are just like you or from your social strata. You will be surprised how similar we all are, and you will become a better and more positive person by interacting with different people. Remember, there are people with negative energy. Limit your interactions with these people. They are not good for your mental health.

Fun

Fun is one of the best things to have. Get out there and do things. Fun activities reduce stress, which affects your mental health, which in turn affects your physical health.

G

Goals

Humans need goals. Never stop trying to achieve something. Having goals gives you hope and something to look forward to. Having goals will force you to meet people, which can result in new, positive relationships with others, which will be a benefit to your mental health.

Take lessons in things. Write a book, make music, play on a team, take a class, join a group, or find a hobby. Turn off the television and computer, stop sitting, and get out there and do something.

Greed

(This is one of the <u>Three Poisons of the Mind</u>-*see also "Hate" on p. 27 and "Ignorance" on p. 31.)*

Greed is probably one of the greatest human impulses in the capitalistic world we live in. In most cases, greed will diminish your mental and moral clarity, sometimes completely. When you are under its influence, you may make poor choices that may not be the best for your mental or physical health. More often than not, greed results in negative consequences to you and your loved ones, because it has the capability to consume your entire existence.

H

Hate

(This is one of the <u>Three Poisons of the Mind</u>-*see also "Greed" on p. 25 and "Ignorance" on p. 31.)*

Learn not to hate. No good comes from it. It will have a disastrous effect on your mental and moral clarity and potentially lead you to bad choices. Moreover, since hate is such a strong emotion, it will increase your stress levels, thus compromising your mental health.

Helpful

Helping others is perhaps one of the most noble and mentally healthy things you can do. Donating money to charitable causes is wonderful, but real satisfaction comes when you actually get out there and do something to help someone, even if it is as simple as just taking someone out for a cup of coffee to discuss a problem.

Hobbies

It is important to have outside interests besides your work and family. Hobbies provide an important mental break for your mind.

Honest

Honesty is the one virtue that will keep you in good standing with your friends, and good things will happen for you as a result. Being deceptive will eventually come back to haunt you, if not directly, then indirectly through bad karma.

Household Cleaning Products/ Beauty Products/Chemicals, etc.

There are a plethora of household products, beauty products, and other items that contain various chemicals and substances that human tissues should not be exposed to. Remember this axiom: *Just because it is legal does not mean it is safe.* Also note that this rule applies to food and beverages.

Do not assume that just because something is for sale that it is safe for you to use on your body or to be in contact with. The fact that some government agencies or studies say something is safe does not mean it actually is. This has been shown time and time again and with food, prescription pills, vitamins, chemicals, and many other types of substances that poison the body.

Foreign substances (together with being in an acidic condition) can and do contribute to cancer formation, neurological problems, and a host of other problems. It can take many years, but the more you damage your cells, the more likely you are to end up sick and unhealthy. Toxins in the body can build up for years before you have problems.

Humble

If you brag or feel the need to talk about something you got or did merely for the sake of validating yourself, you are only lowering your self-worth. Your goodness comes from the seeds that your sow and the help you give others.

I

Ignorance

(This is one of the <u>Three Poisons of the Mind</u>-*see also "Greed" on p. 25 and "Hate" on p. 27.*)

It is easy to be critical, demeaning, and nonchalant when it concerns other people. Try to see things from *other people's perspectives*. People are a product of every experience they have had—from the day they were born to that very day you encounter them now.

Being ignorant of other people's perspectives makes you a narrow-minded person. This in turn makes you more likely to be negative, thus affecting your mental health.

Look forward to interacting with others. You can learn from them, and they can learn from you. It will make you a more full, complete, and happy person.

J

Justice

The purpose of justice is to restore fairness and equality when a person has not been treated properly under the law, and as a result of that conduct the person has suffered or lost something. There is no nobler cause than helping someone who has been wronged by the government, corporations, or other people. Volunteer to help a person achieve justice. This will be a great benefit to your mental well-being, self-accomplishment, and the human condition in general.

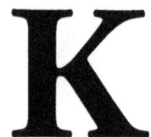

Kindness

Be kind to all people, regardless of what you may think of them. Kindness promotes positive energy that will come back to you in other ways. Being kind helps create a positive mental mood.

L

Laughter

Laughter causes the release of hormones that elevate your mental mood. Your mental mood is deeply tied into your physical well-being.

Love

We all need to feel loved. Some people strive to obtain false love through hollow accomplishments—celebrity, photo opportunities, and the like. People who do this are only setting themselves up for eventual internal disappointment and depression (as history has shown over and over), because these types of activities do not create true love. True love comes only from the people around you who form positive, symbiotic relationships with you. Think about the people with whom you form relationships. Love will flow from them, whether they are spouses, family members, or friends.

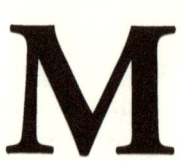

Meat

Many forms of meat can cause your body to become acidic, which leads to a state that is conducive to cell mutation and cancer. Overcooked meat is carcinogenic. Barbecuing cookbooks may be popular, but lots of cooked meat and vegetables with blackened particles on them are unhealthy and carcinogenic.

Many animals in captivity are fed artificially. The feeds and supplements given to many animals, such as chickens, cows, and even fish, are processed nutrition that is carcinogenic, which may instigate cell mutation and thus cancer.

Meat is protein. Too much protein is not healthy and promotes cancer, elevated cholesterol, and digestion problems, among other things.

Meditation

Meditation is an activity that will reduce your stress and thus bolster your physical health. Meditation is an activity, like exercise, that you should try to incorporate into your daily routine. Like water for the physical body, calmness and a lack of stress are the balm for mental health.

Money

Whether you realize it or not, an obsession about acquiring more money will likely add to your stress and corrupt you mentally. Unfortunately, we live in a capitalistic world, one in which the economy is largely based on consumers continually buying "things" that the advertising world tries to convince us we need.

Here's the bottom line: Don't be obsessed with money and material things. In your work, do what you enjoy, and try to help people in the process. If money comes from that, then use it in a good way that enriches your life and the lives of others. (See the related section on "Greed" on p. 25, one of the Three Poisons of the Mind.)

Music

Music is one of the greatest gifts of mankind, and it does wonders for the soul. Embrace all kinds of real music (not artificial), because it provides a natural, healthful rhythm to your body. If you are able to, learn how to play an instrument. It will make your life fuller and more complete and lead to new experiences.

N

Nature

Nature is another one of the greatest gifts to mankind. Embrace it, whether you are walking in the woods, breathing in the salty air of the ocean, or viewing the vistas from the top of a mountain. Visual wonders are good for reducing stress and help you maintain a clearer, healthier mind.

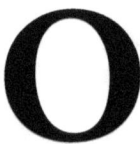

Optimistic

There is always hope. Be positive in all that you do. The undulating rhythms of life are such that there will always be hills and valleys. Look up as you are in a valley, for things will become bright again—they always do. Sometimes, however, it just takes longer. Remember that you have the ability to change your physical and mental habits, so you can become optimistic whenever you desire.

P

Peaceful

Being peaceful means many things to many different people. However, generally speaking, your mental health and stress level will greatly benefit from trying your best to maintain a non-confrontational, non-violent approach to events and people. Reacting to things in any way other than a peaceful one will contribute to your stress not only during the event, but a considerable time thereafter as well. Replaying a stressful event in your mind creates chemical reactions in the brain that are not conducive to good health.

Poisons of the Mind

Hate, greed, and ignorance are the Three Poisons of the Mind that create negative feelings, which definitely affect your physical health, due to the close relationship that exists between the physical body and the mind. (See the respective sections on the these mind poisons, i.e., "Hate", "Greed", and "Ignorance", for more information on each.)

Positive

It is just as easy to have a positive mindset as it is to have a negative one. Your negative thoughts come from the images, thoughts, and words of others. Do not let anyone corrupt your mental clarity and inherent goodness.

Possessions

Possessions are merely substitutes for many things. They will not bring you happiness. After the initial high of a new, allegedly great possession, the appeal will wear off. Owning material possessions does not bring long-lasting happiness. Happiness comes from your relationships with friends and family members, the love you possess in your life, and your moral and ethical strength. (See the related sections of "Greed" on p. 25 and "Money" on p. 40.)

Prescriptions

All prescription drugs have side effects. Just because the FDA or any other agency, medical group, or study approves of a drug, does not mean it is safe. History has shown this to be the case time and time again.

Many drugs on the market are not necessary to take in many situations. The billion-dollar pharmaceutical industry is constantly coming up with drugs for anything and everything, giving them to doctors in order to push them on people, in conjunction with advertising campaigns that tell people why they supposedly need to take a certain pill.

If you eat well and properly maintain a healthy lifestyle, in general, you will not need to take prescription drugs. For example, the idea that some people have high blood pressure or high cholesterol *naturally* is not accurate in many cases.

Health problems such as high blood pressure and high cholesterol, as well as many other conditions that humans can be afflicted with are, for the most part, related to eating habits and lifestyle choices. Some people can eat more "bad" foods earlier in life without them having an adverse effect on their blood pressure, cholesterol, or other body functions (though, eventually, it will affect their health). Humans are not created equal in this way.

You need to eat based on your particular genetic makeup. There is no "one-size-fits-all" approach when it comes to diet. This is why diet books don't work for everyone in the same way.

If there is any way you can wean yourself off of a prescription drug that you don't need, you should do so. Don't think of popping pills as a panacea for all problems, physical or mental. See if there is some way to eliminate use of the drug.

In addition, remain mindful of the side effects and possible damage to your body's tissues from taking prescription medications. Side effects and tissue damage can end up outweighing any claimed benefit of the drug.

Q

Querist

(one who asks questions)

Always ask questions about things you do not know about. Learning is a great gift given to humans, and it is squandered by many people.

Learning and continuing to educate yourself are things that make you a better person. Don't always accept what you are told by governments, corporations, and the news media, all of which, on many occasions, typically have an agenda that may not be in your best interest.

Research and investigate for yourself as you pursue knowledge. Spreading that knowledge thereafter is something that can improve the human condition.

R

Rest

Rest is one of the most important physical functions of the human body. Not having enough rest puts your body in a physical state that is susceptible to disease and sickness. Sleeping, resting, and napping are critical to good physical and mental health. A constant state of being tired or fatigued also leads to sadness and depression because of the chemical reactions taking place in the brain.

S

Sex

Sex is incredibly important. It helps keep you youthful and vibrant. A lack of sex can cause your body to atrophy and become "older." Make time for sex with your mate as often as you can. It will reduce stress. It is also a physical activity that is mentally beneficial, releasing hormones that bolster your overall health.

Simplification

Our modern day lives are frittered away with endless obligations, events, scheduling, and other things that just are not important to the daily human condition. Try as best you can to simplify and to do only what really matters. Don't be afraid to say no to certain people or events. Trying to do too much only adds stress to your life, which will eventually affect your physical health.

Sitting

(being sedentary)

The human animal was not designed to spend endless hours sitting. Thus, a lot of sitting at work or at home in front of the television or computer is unhealthy. These activities promote lower metabolism, and they also can affect the ability to get a good night's sleep. Keep this in mind whenever you are sitting. Standing is better, and you should keep moving as often as you can.

Sleep

The requisite hours of sleep are important for your overall health. A lack of sleep can make one susceptible to disease and sickness. Your body's hormones and systems need a normal sleep cycle in order to keep the body healthy.

The human animal was designed to nap during the day too; our modern life cycle of working and only sleeping at night is unhealthy. Additionally, the human animal was *not* designed to be up at night.

Staying up at night repeatedly, whether it is for work or television, denies your body the ability to heal itself and create hormones that are necessary to battling sickness and disease. Sleeping during the day *does not* make up for this loss. It goes against the natural sleep cycle your body was designed to operate under.

Physical activity during the day will promote a healthful sleep. Once evening comes, you should avoid anything that stimulates the body, and this includes physical activity, mental stress, eating, television, and a host of other things. They are not conducive to good sleep, and they are the primary reasons many people have problems sleeping.

Stress

Besides your diet, this is probably the second most important item to your overall health. Stress affects your physical health and weakens your immune system. Determine the stressors in your life and figure out ways to eliminate or reduce them as much as possible.

Make choices that will not add stress to your life, but reduce it. The combination of a mentally stressed body and an acidic condition creates a much higher likelihood of your body becoming sick and/or diseased.

T

Television

Turn it off and start reading. You need to stimulate your mind. Reading will do a lot more than television ever will. Also, unless you are only watching television, try not to leave it on whenever you're around. Television provides an auditory and visual stimulation, and it creates a mental overload in your brain when you are trying to do other things, because it is distracting. This will affect your mental well-being and increase your stress level.

Time

(as it relates to eating)

The time of day that you eat and what you do after that are both important. Eating and then sitting around doing nothing, or worse, going to sleep, is a poor behavior that contributes to obesity and unhealthiness. Eating close to bedtime and anytime thereafter is unhealthy.

Eat dinner as early as possible to allow your body to properly digest food. Also, eat slowly, not quickly. There is a disconnect between the human stomach and the brain. As a result, people tend to overeat, which means your body could have too many calories to burn, calories that are then stored as fat.

Travel

Man's bond with Earth comes from his relationship with nature and going to new places. Always endeavor to seek out new places every year.

This is not only to experience the greatness of Earth's many amazing and beautiful locations but also to experience different cultures of people. It will make you a better person.

Narrow-mindedness comes from always staying in the same place, seeing the same people, listening to the same thoughts and ideas, and not experiencing new places and cultures.

True

Be true to yourself . . . always. Pursue the things that interest you. Good things will come from that.

U

Understanding

Try to see things from the perspective of others. Doing so will prevent you from having negative thoughts, feelings, and emotions toward other people. Negativity only brings negative energy back to you.

Negative energy and negative thoughts add to your mental stress. This in turn affects your physical health. Besides, mental stress weakens your body's natural ability to fight sicknesses and diseases.

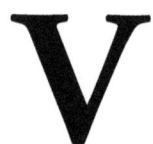

Veracity

Be honest with yourself and others in everything that you do and say. Dishonesty in anything will come back to haunt you, which will add to your stress levels, thus endangering your physical health.

Vitamins

(and supplements)

All of your vitamins and other nutrients should come from fruits, nuts, beans, and vegetables (i.e., the healthy things you eat). If you eat the correct foods, you should not have to take vitamins and supplements.

Vitamins and supplements are part of a huge, corporate, money-making culture that makes billions of dollars convincing people that they need to pop these pills and supplements. Many of them also contain substances that are toxic to your body and that can build up in your tissues, which may eventually lead to sickness and disease.

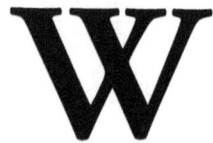

Walking

This is the best exercise you can ever do. The human animal was designed to walk in the quest for food and survival. Walking generates positive hormones that will elevate your mental mood. This activity also will provide a simple and effective means of burning calories and help prevent the body from atrophying from inactivity.

Water

This is the only thing that your body was *ever* designed to drink. *Every other kind of beverage* (with the exception of certain completely natural juices) *contributes to making* your body more acidic, thus promoting the development of sickness and disease.

Water aids your body in flushing the toxins that come from the wrong foods, chemicals, and other substances that damage cells. Failing to drink enough water will cause your body to remain acidic, dehydrated, and unhealthy. Water is like oil in a car engine. If you do not have enough or use other fluids instead, your body will eventually decay and break down.

Many people constantly walk around in a dehydrated state. In most cases, they are not even aware that they are dehydrated, because the human animal is not very good at determining when it needs water. The bottom line is that you shouldn't wait to drink water until you feel "thirsty".

Remember that sugared drinks are carcinogenic. If your genes are such that you are more prone to cancer, too many sugared drinks could increase the odds of your cells mutating and turning into cancer cells.

Weight

Everyone hopefully knows by now that excess weight contributes to poor physical and emotional health. The most important factors of weight are what you eat and drink, when you eat, how much you eat, how much you are sedentary, and the amount of stress you have.

If you fail to eat the correct foods in the proper ways, you will likely gain excess weight. Exercise does not eliminate the problem, which is why you see lots of overweight people who exercise. This is because they eat the wrong foods, eat too much, and eat at night too close to bedtime.

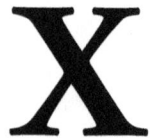

Xenodochial

This means being hospitable to strangers. Remember the Golden Rule: *Do unto others as you would have them do unto you.*

Y

Yes

Say yes to things you might not always want to do. New experiences enhance your mental health. Experiencing new things is extremely important to your mental health. As a result of this approach, you will meet new people and form new relationships and bonds.

The human animal needs interaction with others to be mentally healthy. Don't fall into the same boring routine of doing the same things all the time and going to the same places when you travel. Mental health has a direct correlation to your physical health.

z

Zen

Understand the concept of mindfulness, which is a Buddhist concept that details how not to be concerned with the future or worried about the past. Live in the moment and concentrate on that. This will reduce stress and make you a happier person.

Appendix

The General Health Formula:

$$[(\text{Diet}^2) \times (\text{Physical Activity})] \div [(\text{Stress} + \text{External Environment})]$$

Note: This is an abstract formula. There are no numbers to plug into the sections. It is just something to consider when you are analyzing your lifestyle.

1. Diet is "squared," because this is the most important factor in your overall health.

2. Your diet factor (how good it is) is then multiplied by your physical activity.

3. This left side of the equation is then divided by the right side of the equation (the negative factors, which include your stress and your living/working environment).